HEALING THE HEALER

HEALING THE HEALER

POSITIVE AFFIRMATIONS FOR THE HEALING PROFESSIONS

Dr Hendrik B. Lai
MBA, MS-Management, Grad.Cert. -
Organizational Leadership, BDS, CM,
CPMgr, FCMI, FAIM, FInstAM, FIIDM,
AFCHSM

Mosen Fofel Publishing, Sheboygan, WI

COPYRIGHT

The information presented in this work solely and fully represents the views of the author as of the date of publication. Any omission, or potential misrepresentation of any persons or companies is entirely unintentional. As a result of changing information, condition or contexts, the author reserves the right to alter content at their sole discretion and impunity.

This work is for informational purposes only and while every attempt has been made to verify the accuracy of the information contained herein, the author assumes no responsibility for errors, inaccuracies and omissions. Each person has unique needs and this work cannot take these individual differences into account.

This work is copyright © 2017 by Hendrik Lai with all rights reserved.

Published by Mosen Fofel Publishing, Sheboygan WI USA.

ISBN 978-0-6481100-0-2

ABOUT THE AUTHOR

Dr Hendrik B. Lai is a practicing dental surgeon and entrepreneur. He is also an experienced business consultant and an Adjunct Senior Lecturer at the College of Medicine and Dentistry at James Cook University. He is a founder and principal consultant at Schleining, Eldred, Lai and Company and serves as a Director of American Pacific Investments.

Hendrik is passionate about patient and practitioner health in regional and rural areas and has been featured by dozens of media outlets including the Sydney Morning Herald, ABC, Channel Seven, Channel TEN, WIN and Australia Network. He has spoken extensively on health economics, strategy and health care access issues.

Hendrik and his wife, Sylvia, are the proud parents of Helena and Ethan and reside in Sheboygan County, Wisconsin.

CONTENTS

INTRODUCTION	3
GIVE YOUR DAY A POSITIVE START	15
INCREASE YOUR SELF-CONFIDENCE	19
INCREASE YOUR CREATIVITY	23
OVERCOME YOUR FEARS	27
COPING WITH THE LOSS OF A PATIENT	33
DEALING WITH FAILURE	39
THE ROAD TO HAPPINESS	45
OPTIMIZE YOUR PERFORMANCE	49
INCREASE YOUR TIME MANAGEMENT SKILLS	53
ADAPTING TO CHANGE	57
END YOUR DAY WITH PEACE AND LOVE	61
CONCLUSION	65

INTRODUCTION

It's no secret that stress and health care go hand-in-hand, indeed recent media reports have shone a spotlight on stress in the healing professions and its at times tragic consequences. The seemingly endless years of study with your nose to the grindstone, followed by highly competitive internships are just the beginning.

When you finally enter your chosen profession there is the busy clinical environment, with the long hours of dedication and sacrifice - and all of the blood, sweat, and tears you put into saving lives and helping others in need.

It would be far from being cliché if I said "a healer's life is not easy." Healers find themselves confronted with many challenges during the course of their working day. Needless to say, as these challenges mound up throughout the course of the day, they can breed more stress than is healthy, even in the hardiest of souls.

It can seem that as a healer you are destined to be buried under a mountain of stress from the moment you graduate from college:

- You are more than likely to have a significant level of debt from student loans after you graduate from your professional school. This immediately places a large financial stress on you and can leave you with a lot worry and anxiety about the future as you walk the tightrope of doing the right thing by your patients with the financial imperative of servicing your loans.

- You work long, often thankless hours that more often than not extend into the most unsociable hours of the day.

- You are constantly under pressure from your family and friends to dedicate more time to them, but by the nature of your work, you cannot always be available. Even your time off is not fully your own. Being "on call" you may get summoned back into work at a moment's notice.

- You have to deal with people from all walks of life many of who will be in distress. Some people will be an absolute pleasure to treat. Others will make you want to pull your hair out.

- You have to make fast and effective decisions often in volatile situations with ambiguous information. This can result in decision fatigue leaving you feeling exhausted and overwhelmed.

- You will generally be surrounded by more negativity in your work environment than other professions, because for the most part happy and healthy people do not go to their doctor's office or the hospital.

- You are surrounded by colleagues, patients and relatives all of whom look to you for guidance and may place exceedingly high expectations on you.

I'm sure that some of the above stress inducing situations faced by healers will resonate with you. The above list is not intended to be exhaustive as this would be an entire book in itself. Instead it is designed to showcase the stark reality of just some of the stresses you have to deal with every day that you may not even have been aware of.

In this book, I am offering you positive self-affirmations that will help you be your best everyday and in everyway. Being a healer myself, I understand that time is a decaying resource – every second that passes is a second that can never be recovered. For your convenience, I have indexed in the table of contents positive affirmations covering the following situations:

- Kick-starting a busy day
- Increasing your self-confidence
- Increasing your creativity
- Overcoming your fear and anxiety
- Finding inner-peace
- Coping with the loss of patients
- Dealing with failure
- Optimizing your performance
- Increasing your time management skills
- Adapting to change
- Ending your day in a calm and relaxed way

Why Positive Affirmations?

Simply because they work. Positive affirmations have been scientifically proven to help people from all walks of life. There has been some very powerful research that reveals evidence of changes in brain activity in people who practice positive self-affirmations on a regular basis.

The power of positive affirmations is by no means a modern phenomenon. French psychologist and pharmacist Emile Coué first analyzed the effects of positive affirmations on the brain nearly 100 years ago. He is credited for his philosophy of "every day in every way I am getting better and better."

Coué believed that concentrated attention created a new thought pattern in his clients enabling them to turn their thoughts into reality. He called his method "Conscious Autosuggestion". He suggested that these affirmations should be practiced in a quiet place for at least 10 to 20 minutes each day. According to Coué the best times to practice affirmations were either when you wake up or when you go to sleep.

A more recent scientific study conducted at the University of Pennsylvania by Christopher Cascio sheds some more light on the effectiveness of positive affirmations. Dr. Cascio and his team used magnetic resonance imaging to investigate the changes that took place in the brains of people who practiced these kinds of affirmations.

What they found was that self-affirmation techniques created a higher level of activity in the areas of the brain responsible for behavioral changes by creating a new set of neuronal connections. This was particularly noticeable in the ventral striatum and the ventral medial prefrontal cortex. These parts of the brain are responsible for reward and "self" related thinking. Essentially what the researchers found was that positive affirmations about the future caused the brain to rewire itself to expect the affirmation to be fulfilled.

Furthermore, research conducted at Carnegie Mellon University found that positive affirmations could protect people from the damaging effects of stress. What this study found was that even a brief affirmation exercise was enough to eliminate the deleterious effects of chronic stress on problem-solving performance.

The take away message is that there is a significant body of scientific evidence that supports the effectiveness of positive self-affirmations particularly in reducing stress and improving performance.

Implementing self-affirmations does not have a steep learning curve. As you first embark on using self-affirmations, I recommend following Coué's suggested protocol of undertaking the affirmations on waking in the morning and before retiring for the evening. I suggest following this protocol for at least the first two weeks or until it becomes easy for you to maintain concentration on the affirmations without too much effort.

Once you start to become more comfortable and familiar with the process of self-affirmation, you can practice the process anytime during the day, whenever you feel the need for it.

You will instinctively know when you are ready to move on to the next step. You can apply these affirmations not only in the morning or at night, but also before or after surgery or other stressful procedures, or anytime you feel stressed and just need a little boost from your inner cheerleader.

When you know you are likely have a particularly difficult day, it is useful to take the time to write down three or four positive affirmations on a slip of paper for easy reference. Put this slip of paper in a shirt or blouse pocket. When you need them most they will be within easy reach. So take a quiet minute during your day to read from your list of affirmations to help focus yourself and set yourself in the right frame of mind.

These positive self-affirmations are not intended to be a replacement or substitute for professional help. Indeed, they are designed to augment your own capabilities and support professional assistance. Remember, there is no need to suffer in silence and I would encourage you to make use of all the resources, internal and external, available to you.

Remember that the body follows the mind and you can change your mindset when you set your heart and mind to it!

GIVE YOUR DAY A POSITIVE START

The path of the healer is not the path most travelled. You work long hours to heal others and find solutions to their often complex problems. You are at higher risk of becoming exhausted both mentally and physically, much more so than almost any other profession. Since you spend the day handling other people's lives and their health, it is important to give your day the energetic and uplifting start that it needs.

When you begin your workday with a well-primed and better-organized brain, you will find it easier to deal with your tasks. It will not only help you, but it will also help your team, your patients, and your family too. Make these affirmations a part of your miracle morning, repeating them while you are still in bed. Then rise and greet the day with positivity and clarity!

- I feel the positive energy flowing into me like a shining light from the universe.
- I choose calmness over anxiety, and I let the anxiety leave my body.
- I have everything I need within me.
- I choose to be strong and positive.
- I have the power to deal with the problems I will face today and every day.
- I will not let stress control me and affect my actions.
- I have unlimited potential.
- I make good changes in people's lives.

- I am in charge of my decisions and I choose positivity and motivation.
- I know how to motivate others and myself.
- I am ready to face the day and whatever it brings my way.
- I am grateful for my life.
- I am grateful for my job.
- I love my job because it gives me the opportunity to change people's lives for the better.
- I am a good example for my colleagues.
- I have all the support I need from my family and my friends.
- I am healthy both physically and mentally.
- I trust my inner thoughts and my intuition.
- Today is filled with possibilities and new beginnings.
- I have an open heart and an open mind.
- I am unique and I do not compare myself to others.

- I work on myself to get better than I was yesterday.
- I woke up as a better person this morning.
- I know each day is a gift and I honor my life and my body knowing this.
- I am patient with myself and I am patient with others.
- I know how to listen to others.
- I accept myself and respect myself.
- I am starting my day with a good mood and I want to help others get and feel better too.
- I trust myself and my colleagues and my patients trust me too.
- I always want the best for my patients.
- I give out love with everything I say and do.
- I have the courage to begin my day.

INCREASE YOUR SELF-CONFIDENCE

Self-confidence is vital for healers and those that support them in the care of patients and their loved ones. There are many times during your day when you will find yourself in situations where you will need to make quick decisions, with incomplete information, all while your whole team is looking to you for leadership and hanging on your every word for guidance.

As much as you may hate to admit it, you are human and you will have doubts and uncertainties like anyone else.

The pressure of the situation and the internal pressure you put on yourself can easily make matters worse and cause you to question your decisions. Making you second-guess everything you know and feel about yourself and your abilities. These self-affirmations are for you to use to increase your self-esteem before stress kicks in, so you are already equipped with what you need to bolster your mental immunity.

- I let go of all uncertainties and I let go of my shyness.
- I am accustomed to dealing with all kinds of situations and I have the knowledge to deal with them.
- I have the confidence I need to make the right decisions.
- My team trusts me and knows that I am doing my best.

- Self-confidence is like a second nature to me.
- I am energetic and I can make decisions fast.
- I can solve the problems with ease in a calm way.
- I focus on solutions and I can see the best possible outcomes.
- I can adapt to changes easily and I do not let change scare me.
- Challenges are an essential part of my job and I welcome them every day, every minute.
- I always see the good in others and they see the good in me too.
- I approach everyone with acceptance and love.
- The more confidence I have, the better my team and my patients feel.
- My patients trust me and they know I think of them.
- I know how to get out of unpleasant situations with confidence.
- My patients know I love them and I care about them.

- I have the knowledge and the talent I need to help others feel and get better.
- I deserve to be happy.
- I deserve to be successful.
- I know how to forgive others and move on in a positive direction.
- I am dedicated to my patients.
- I know how to listen to my patients and their needs.
- I communicate with my team openly.
- I focus on my patients and their needs and they know that I do.
- I am not insecure.
- I am not shy or timid.
- My skills increase every day, day by day.
- I know how to handle the most stressful medical conditions.
- I know how to cure people and people trust me.
- Helping others is what makes me happy.

INCREASE YOUR CREATIVITY

We know that analytical thinking is a must for a healer, but you also need ensure that you nurture your creative thinking to maintain a healthy balance. There are times when we all find ourselves clogged creatively. Getting bogged down in daily tasks and the stress that comes with them can mean that we don't give enough time to nurturing our "right brain" resulting in a lack of creativity and inner balance.

As a healer, you know that achieving a wholeness of mind and body is important and perhaps you are looking for ways to unwind your brain by doing things that will give your creative side a turbo boost.

Having a hobby outside of your profession will relieve your stress and can boost your self-esteem at the same time. You will feel more connected to your spiritual side as you give freely of yourself and you will raise your outlook to a more positive plane.

When you increase your creativity, you will increase your motivation. When you increase your motivation, you will increase your performance in almost every aspect of your life. Here are some positive affirmations to help you awaken your creative mind.

- I am a creative person.
- I am open-minded and I am a free thinker.

- I welcome new ideas both at my job and in my personal life.
- My creativity flows like a river.
- I have dreams and I know how to achieve them.
- I find inspiration very easily in everywhere I look.
- My patients inspire me to do good things.
- My creativity is limitless and it inspires my patients too.
- My creativity is increasing every day.
- I always come up with new ideas and I always see new perspectives.
- The universe gives me creative energy.
- I inspire others to find their creativity too.
- My imagination is powerful.
- I appreciate my inner child because it reminds me of who I really am.
- I am peaceful and at ease.
- I make my patients feel peaceful and at ease.
- I make my colleagues feel peaceful and at ease.

- I am sincere and it shows through my words and actions.
- I know how to make others happy.
- The universe inspires me to create new things every day.
- Creative ideas find me wherever I go.
- I am not afraid of expressing myself.
- I let others express themselves and they feel comfortable around me.
- I am ready to share my ideas with others.
- I love listening to other people's ideas because I always learn new things.
- I love surprises and I love surprising others equally.
- When I am creative, I become a better healer.
- I never doubt my creative powers.
- I have the mental power to overcome creativity blocks.
- I will eliminate all negative thoughts and emotions.
- I choose to use my mental power to create good things.

OVERCOME YOUR FEARS

As a healer, you'll likely find yourself confronted with situations that can strike fear into even the hardiest of souls. You may have to deal with highly contagious illnesses like the Ebola virus. Maybe a fear of contracting the virus or a similarly nasty infection and unintentionally passing it to your loved ones might keep you up at night.

Having these fears are valid and to an extent necessary to prevent foolhardiness. However, if these fears gain control, they might cause you to second guess yourself and your decisions. Did you do the right thing for that patient? What if you had done this, instead of that? What if the decision you made will result in more serious complications?

Sometimes you have to take calculated, necessary risks because you work in a volatile, uncertain, complex and ambiguous environment where there is often no easy clear-cut answer or solution. Sometimes you have to choose between the lesser of two evils when deciding on the optimal course of care for your patients.

Bearing such a heavy burden on your shoulders will take its toll sooner or later. Much of the time, it is our fear of failure that causes us to sabotage our own selves. We know that the fear of failure saps motivation and lowers self-esteem. You can use these affirmations by themselves or use them together with self-confidence affirmations to kick fear to the curb since fear and self-esteem are closely tied.

- I am ready to take action.
- I am ready to make important decisions bravely.
- I can handle problems with a clear head.
- I am free from fear of failure; I do not let fear take over me.
- I am confident in my decisions and I take action with self-confidence.
- I choose to push my boundaries to be better at my job.
- I accept challenges.
- I am not afraid of illnesses.
- I am not afraid of getting sick because I live healthily.
- I know how to protect myself and my family.
- I know how to protect my team and my patients.
- Even if I fail, I know how to get up and try again.
- I do not let failure bring me down.

- My courage inspires my patients and my team.
- I learn from my mistakes.
- I learn from others' mistakes because I pay attention to others always.
- I become more and more fearless each day.
- It is easy for me to make important decisions on a short notice.
- I know how to focus on my patients and I know how to help them.
- Setbacks don't scare me; I see them as life lessons.
- I am positive and I radiate positive energy to my patients.
- I can see the fearful thoughts and emotions leave my mind and my body.
- I will not let fearful thoughts tighten my chest today.
- I am overcoming my fears one by one each day.
- I have peace of mind knowing I always do the best I can.
- I invite love and peace into my life.

- I choose to believe in myself and my abilities.
- I am not afraid of injuries.
- I have faith in myself.

COPING WITH THE LOSS OF A PATIENT

As Benjamin Franklin famously said "nothing can be said to be certain, except death and taxes." In the healing arts, you may be exposed to the inevitability of death on a daily basis. Much as you might try, you cannot save everyone and sooner or later, you will find yourself confronting this harsh reality.

There is the loss of an old favorite patient, the loss of a young patient in the prime of their lives, and sometimes the loss of an infant or a newborn baby who is taken at the very beginning of life's journey. No matter what your patient's age is, it can be incredibly difficult to cope with the loss of a patient. Even though this is something you may be trained to deal with, the fact is, it is a human life that has been lost.

As a healer, not only do you feel a responsibility towards your patients, you feel a responsibility towards the loved ones the patient leaves behind. Everyone wants answers - everyone wants to know "why and how?"

You may find yourself asking if there really was nothing else you could possibly have done for this patient to save their life and ease their pain. You may find yourself tasked with making the most difficult of executive decisions that cuts to the very essence of life and what it takes to sustain it.

Our society teaches us to internalize how we feel – the thoughts and feelings of a surgeon or physician are not always spoken freely. There is often no immediate counseling for this; there is little time to dwell on this pain because you have to move on quickly to help others – as the saying goes, "life goes on". Other patients are waiting for you and expecting you to help them. Your team expects you to lead them and work with them effectively no matter the situation. These affirmations may help you better cope with the loss of a patient.

- I am confident that I do the best I can to help my patients.
- I know that sometimes things might not go as planned and I am prepared to face it.
- I know that I cannot save every life.
- I know that my patients trust me.
- I know that my team trusts me and approves my decisions.
- I choose to not let the grief overpower me so I can help others as they need.

- I know the universe will guide me in the right direction.
- I know that the universe will give me the strength I need to cope with a loss.
- I know how to let go of sadness and grief.
- I am thankful for the opportunities my job gives me.
- I am thankful to know my patients and to help them.
- I am willing to accept the things I cannot change.
- I know people love me and they have confidence in me.
- I love everyone equally and I help them equally.
- I have compassion for everyone.
- I treasure life and health.
- I appreciate the things I have.
- I value life and the people that come into my life.
- I am willing to release my sorrow and pain.

- I am relaxed and I am ready to move on.
- I will take care of myself so I can take care of others.
- My life has a purpose and I will work towards it.
- This will pass.
- I can still make good decisions even if I feel sad or bad.
- I am stronger than I was before.
- I learn from my experiences and I let them make me a better healer.

DEALING WITH FAILURE

As in every job, things can and will go wrong, taking a turn for the worse despite our best efforts. As a healer, you will feel pressured to give answers because you are responsible for the wellbeing and lives of others. Failure can take many forms. At its extreme, failure might result in the loss of a patient. Sometimes it may mean that you have made a mistake simply because you are human and as such an imperfect being.

Depending on your field, the seriousness of a mistake can be difficult to deal with. Sometimes the outcome can be trivial - sometimes it can be fatal. There are always unexpected complications you will have to deal with as a healer. You may have the best of intentions, but for one reason or another you might not be as successful as you would like. Sometimes the complications can be caused by technical issues and not be related to patient factors.

Unfortunately, in spite of all the planning in the world, there is no way to completely avoid complications. This is a part of the job that you will never be able to fully mitigate, no matter how experienced and careful you are.

What would you do? Do you blame someone else for your actions? Do you bury your pain and pretend it never happened? None of these mindsets will bring you peace. So what can you do? Try reading these affirmations, being as honest as you can with yourself so you can move on with helping and healing others.

- I cannot control everything and I accept the things I cannot change.
- Everything happens for a reason, even if I don't understand it.
- I am not perfect and I never claim to be perfect.
- I am prepared for the complications, but I also know that I cannot control everything.
- I extend compassion and love to myself because I deserve it.
- I do not judge myself because I know I try to do the best I can.
- I do not blame others for my actions. I take full responsibility for my actions, but I do not let them destroy me.
- I will learn from my mistakes and continue to grow.
- If I keep loving myself, I will love my patients too.

- If I show compassion to myself I will feel compassion for my patients too.
- If I make mistakes they are never intentional.
- I accept the difficulties of being a healer.
- I accept that nothing is predictable.
- I choose to stay balanced and healthy.
- I choose to let go of my fears and worries.
- I choose to let go of guilt.
- I will turn bad experiences into positive outcomes for my future.
- I will not let bad experiences affect my future.
- I will not let fear of failure stop my personal and professional growth and development.
- I will not let anxiety stand in my way.
- I am able to continue working and doing better things.
- I overcome failure smoothly.
- I will find a way to get better at what I do.

- I will let go of the past and welcome the future.
- I know my family and my colleagues always have compassion for me.

THE ROAD TO HAPPINESS

As a healer, your life's work is to make the lives of others better. You want them to leave your office or the hospital feeling joyful and happy. You know how to give happiness to others in most cases, but what do you do to find happiness? How do you keep your head above water to survive? How do you find inner peace? As a healer, you know that a happy mind means a healthy body. But in your line of work, you are measured in many different ways.

A patient's satisfaction and happiness is something we all talk about, with more metrics and key performance indicators that measure this than you can poke a stick at. However, we rarely talk about the healer's satisfaction and happiness. Think about your goals and your dreams. Think about the things that make you smile and make you feel love and loved. Use these positive affirmations for self-support.

- I have the right to be happy.
- I deserve happiness and the universe brings me happiness in many different ways.
- I choose happiness over worry and anxiety.
- When I am happy, I make others happy.
- Everyday happiness fills my entire body.
- I am a healer; I touch people's lives. My happiness makes my patients happy too.

- I enjoy my life and everyone and everything in it.
- Getting better at my job makes me happy.
- Seeing my patients get better brings me joy and happiness.
- Happiness comes to me naturally.
- The whole universe conspires to bring me more and more happiness.
- When I think about my future, I feel happiness.
- I am filled with love and kindness.
- I am compassionate, gentle, and thoughtful.
- Everything I need is already within me.
- I am strong enough to create the life I deserve.
- I love myself unconditionally.
- I am open to receive love and kindness.
- I am physically and emotionally strong.
- I am healthy.

- I always choose positive thoughts and let go of negative emotions.

OPTIMIZE YOUR PERFORMANCE

As you transition through your career, you will often find yourself facing tough situations. Sometimes you'll work long hours; sometimes you'll work overnight. Sometimes you'll work for what seems like days on end without a break. There are times that you'll be physically and mentally exhausted and you don't feel you have the energy to perform your duties.

When you are in these situations, this lack of energy might sap your motivation, but more importantly, can detract from your overall performance. However, like the proverbial superhero, when someone needs your help, you have to find ways to quickly recharge your batteries and stand ready to answer the call of duty. Here are some positive affirmations to help give you clarity and energy.

- I am always clear-headed and focused.
- I have the energy to keep going even during the most difficult times.
- I am full of energy both physically and mentally.
- I do not get tired easily.
- The universe fills me with energy.
- I can perform my tasks without getting tired.
- I fall asleep easily and I get enough sleep each day.
- I eat healthy to take care of my body.
- My motivation is always high.
- Every day I am getting more energetic.

- I have an abundance of energy within me and around me.
- I know how to stay healthy.
- Doing my job gives me more and more energy.
- The more I work, the more motivation I find.
- I am in better shape than I ever was.
- I have good endurance and it keeps improving each day.
- I work hard.
- I am in charge of my life.
- I am in control of my thoughts and emotions.
- My family and friends support me in the things I do.
- I am confident and I can overcome any obstacle.
- I am prepared for challenges and changes.
- I work fast.
- I pay attention to everything I have to do for my patients.

INCREASE YOUR TIME MANAGEMENT SKILLS

A sad reality of modern health care is that healers often find themselves moving quickly from one patient to another. Each patient has different needs and each case requires different treatments or collaboration with colleagues. Some cases take more time than others. Paperwork in between patients seems to take up an ever-increasing amount of precious time.

Even if you have good time management skills you might still find it difficult to deal with all of the competing priorities mounded on you. Here are some helpful affirmations for you.

- My time management skills are outstanding.
- I plan things in advance.
- I finish everything on time.
- I am successful because I am good at managing my time.
- I am ready to face unexpected events.
- I won't let surprises and setbacks ruin my daily routine.
- I keep good track of my schedule.
- I always check my calendar before I start my day.
- I have time for everything.
- I am getting better at managing my tasks.
- I know how to set my priorities.
- I always come to work on time.
- I know how to use my time effectively.
- My time is precious.

- I value my time.
- I give enough time to myself.
- I take the time to take care of myself.
- I make time for my family and friends.
- People respect my time management skills.
- I am known for my time management skills.
- I know how to use my time to be productive.
- I know how to use my time to rest and rejuvenate.
- I give myself enough time to sleep.
- I give myself enough time to eat healthily.
- I give myself enough time to take care of my body.
- I respect other people's time.
- I do not take other people's time for granted.
- I am grateful for being organized.

ADAPTING TO CHANGE

As a healer, you already know how important adaptability is. And as a healer, you are most probably already better equipped than most at being adaptable and agile, after all, constant change comes with the territory. Seeing one patient after another under volatile and uncertain conditions. The difficulty of keeping track of an exponentially increasing number of tasks. However, there are many things you can do to adapt to changes smoothly and effectively.

You already have the stamina to move from one case to another with agility. But at the end of the day, you may find yourself running on the smell of an oily rag. You might find yourself confused, distracted and mentally exhausted. You can use the positive affirmations below to help you overcome your feelings of inertia to excel in the dynamic health care environment.

- I welcome changes and I find a positive side in all of them.
- I accept changes as they come.
- I am ready to adapt changes in my life and at work.
- I can change things when I want to.
- I see each day as an exciting opportunity.
- I will take the challenges as they come.
- I let go of the things I cannot change.
- I let go of negative thoughts and emotions.

- Each brings new surprises for me and for others.
- I will overcome each obstacle with ease.
- Changes do not affect my performance - they improve it.
- My team admires my positivity when facing changes and challenges.
- I am thankful for my job.
- I am thankful for the constant changes and challenges, they make me stronger.
- I am kind and compassionate no matter what happens.
- I keep my patience even when things don't go as planned.
- Every patient will bring a new challenge that will help me grow.
- I have the knowledge to solve my problems.
- I have the strength to find solutions to my problems.

END YOUR DAY WITH PEACE AND LOVE

Finally your working day draws to a close. At the end of a long and busy day, you need to wind down before you retire for the day so you can get a restful night's sleep to prepare for the day to come.

Unfortunately, we often find ourselves dwelling on the stresses of the day, our minds racing and not wanting to put aside the thoughts and emotions of the day. You may find your mind starts replaying the day's events over and over again. You may start thinking of certain situation or patients and may question your actions and decisions.

While a degree of reflection is healthy and indeed necessary for personal growth, it is very important for you to relax and put these self-limiting and tiring thoughts aside.

Apart from positive affirmations, there are other things you can do to relax and re-energize in your daily life. You might try to volunteer for a cause that fills you with purpose, you can take the time to exercise, you can practice mindfulness meditation or maybe if the opportunity arises, you can teach young healers as well. But once you are in bed and getting ready to let slumber take you for the night, try repeating these affirmations for a more restful repose.

- I am thankful for everything I have learned today.

- I am thankful for all the new people I have met today.
- I let go of my worries right now.
- I let go of stress and anxiety right now.
- I am ready to relax.
- With each breath I take, sleep fills my body.
- With each breath I exhale, thoughts leave my body.
- I am focused.
- Sleep is waiting for me and I will have a good long sleep tonight.
- I am ready to wind down, and I feel good.
- I am accomplished.
- I have finished all my tasks today.
- I am thankful for my family.
- I am thankful for my life.
- I am healthy.
- I release all tension now.
- My muscles are relaxed.
- I feel like a feather and I am floating peacefully.
- I am ready to sleep.

CONCLUSION

I hope the positive self-affirmations in this book will help you relax and better focus on yourself and your wellbeing. Remember to set aside a specific time for this each day. In the beginning, try to do this at the same time every day so your brain habituates the process and can more efficiently reprogram itself.

You might find it difficult, especially in the beginning, to keep your focus for a long time. It is important not to feel discouraged.

With practice you will become more proficient, and every day the amount of time you will be able to focus without interruption will increase. You will become better at managing your thoughts and emotions and keeping them organized.

After a month or so you will notice the difference. You can then practice these affirmations anytime and anywhere - while sitting and waiting in traffic, between patients, before surgery, or before or after staff meetings. Your body will tell you when it needs this special time. You will know when you need to recharge your batteries or when you need to wind down.

Above all, remain positive. Positivity is important for all of us. To paraphrase Buddha: "The mind is everything. What we think, we become". Believe in yourself and your power to change the things you don't like. Because what you need is already within you. You don't necessarily need to spend money to achieve these things. You only need to believe in yourself and your abilities as a human being.

You are already equipped with all the motivation, and all the strength to get through the toughest experiences. When you are positive, you will see that your inner vision will broaden and it will show you endless possibilities, some of which you didn't know were there before. You have the power to take control of your life.